Eucalyptus Oil

Unleashing the Healing Power of Nature: The Remarkable Benefits and Uses

Dr Max Holden
Copyright@2023

Table of Contents

CHAPTER ONE

Introduction to Eucalyptus Oil

Eucalyptus oil is a natural essential oil that is extracted from the leaves of the eucalyptus tree, which is native to Australia. It has a distinctive aroma and a range of therapeutic properties that have been used for centuries in traditional medicine. This chapter will provide an overview of what eucalyptus oil is, how it is extracted, and its historical use in traditional medicine. We will also highlight the key components of eucalyptus oil that give it its unique healing properties.

What is Eucalyptus Oil?

Eucalyptus oil is a volatile oil that is derived from the leaves of the eucalyptus tree. There are over 700 species of eucalyptus, but the most common species used for oil production is Eucalyptus globulus. The oil is extracted through a process of steam distillation, which involves heating the leaves and collecting the resulting vapor. The oil that is collected is a clear, colorless liquid with a strong, fresh, and medicinal aroma.

Historical Use of Eucalyptus Oil

Eucalyptus has been used for medicinal purposes for centuries. The Aboriginal people of Australia have used eucalyptus leaves to treat wounds, infections, and respiratory ailments for thousands of years. When Europeans arrived in Australia, they quickly recognized the potential of eucalyptus oil and began exporting it to Europe for use in medicine and perfumery.

In the 19th century, eucalyptus oil became popular in Europe as a treatment for respiratory infections, such as tuberculosis and influenza. During World War I, eucalyptus oil was used as an antiseptic to treat wounds and prevent infections. Today, eucalyptus oil is widely used in aromatherapy, as well as in traditional medicine, for its wide range of therapeutic properties.

Key Components of Eucalyptus Oil

Eucalyptus oil contains a range of compounds that give it its unique healing properties. The most abundant component of eucalyptus oil is 1,8-cineole, also known as eucalyptol, which makes up between 70-90% of the oil. Other components include alpha-pinene, limonene, and terpinen-4-ol, all of which contribute to the oil's antimicrobial, anti-inflammatory, and analgesic properties.

The high concentration of 1,8-cineole in eucalyptus oil is responsible for its potent respiratory benefits. When inhaled, eucalyptus oil can help to clear the sinuses, reduce inflammation in the airways, and alleviate symptoms of respiratory infections such as coughs and colds.

In conclusion, eucalyptus oil is a natural essential oil that has been used for centuries for its therapeutic properties. It is extracted from the leaves of the eucalyptus tree through a process of steam distillation and contains a range of compounds, including 1,8-cineole, that give it its unique healing properties. Eucalyptus oil has a long history of use in traditional medicine and is widely used today in aromatherapy and natural remedies for its wide range of health benefits.

CHAPTER TWO

Health Benefits of Eucalyptus Oil

Eucalyptus oil is known for its many health benefits, some of which have been supported by scientific research. In this chapter, we will explore the different ways eucalyptus oil can improve our health.

Respiratory Health Eucalyptus oil is commonly used to relieve respiratory problems, such as coughs, colds, and congestion. The oil contains compounds that help to open up the airways and reduce inflammation, making it easier to breathe. Research has shown that inhaling eucalyptus oil can help to reduce symptoms of asthma and bronchitis.

Anti-Inflammatory Properties Eucalyptus oil has anti-inflammatory properties that make it useful in treating a variety of conditions, such as arthritis and joint pain. These properties are due to the presence of compounds called cineole and limonene, which have been shown to reduce inflammation and pain.

Antiseptic and Antibacterial Properties Eucalyptus oil has powerful antiseptic and antibacterial properties, making it effective in treating skin infections, wounds, and burns. These properties are due to the presence of compounds such as eucalyptol and alpha-terpineol, which have been shown to kill harmful bacteria and prevent infection.

Pain Relief Eucalyptus oil has analgesic properties that make it effective in relieving pain. The oil can be applied topically to the skin or used in massage therapy to alleviate muscle and joint pain. The anti-inflammatory properties of eucalyptus oil also contribute to its pain-relieving effects.

Mental Health Eucalyptus oil has a calming effect on the mind and body, making it useful in reducing stress and anxiety. Inhaling the oil through aromatherapy can help to promote relaxation and improve mood. Additionally, the oil can be used in massage therapy to promote relaxation and reduce tension in the muscles.

Dental Health Eucalyptus oil has been shown to have antimicrobial properties that make it effective in promoting oral health. The oil can be used to treat gum disease, bad breath, and toothaches. It can also be added to toothpaste and mouthwash to improve overall oral hygiene.

In conclusion, eucalyptus oil has a wide range of health benefits that make it a valuable natural remedy. Its anti-inflammatory, analgesic, antiseptic, antibacterial, and calming properties make it useful in treating a variety of conditions and promoting overall health and well-being. However, it is important to use eucalyptus oil safely and consult a healthcare professional before using it to treat any specific health condition.

Practical Uses for Eucalyptus Oil

Eucalyptus oil is a versatile and multipurpose oil that can be used for a wide range of practical purposes. In this chapter, we will explore some of the most common and effective uses for eucalyptus oil, including aromatherapy, household cleaning, and skincare.

Aromatherapy with Eucalyptus Oil Aromatherapy is the use of essential oils to promote physical and emotional well-being. Eucalyptus oil is a popular essential oil used in aromatherapy due to its refreshing and uplifting scent. Some ways to incorporate eucalyptus oil into aromatherapy include:

1. Diffusing eucalyptus oil in a diffuser or adding a few drops to a bowl of hot water and inhaling the steam for respiratory benefits.
2. Adding a few drops of eucalyptus oil to a warm bath for a soothing and relaxing experience.
3. Adding a few drops of eucalyptus oil to a carrier oil and using it for a relaxing massage.

Household Cleaning with Eucalyptus Oil

Eucalyptus oil has powerful antibacterial and antiviral properties that make it an effective natural cleaner. Here are some ways to use eucalyptus oil for household cleaning:

1. Add a few drops of eucalyptus oil to a spray bottle of water to create a natural disinfectant for surfaces such as countertops, sinks, and toilets.

2. Add a few drops of eucalyptus oil to your laundry detergent to help kill

bacteria and freshen up clothes and linens.

3. Mix eucalyptus oil with vinegar and water for an all-purpose cleaner that can be used on floors, windows, and mirrors.

Skincare with Eucalyptus Oil

Eucalyptus oil has a cooling and soothing effect on the skin, making it an ideal ingredient for skincare products. Here are some ways to use eucalyptus oil in your skincare routine:

- Mix a few drops of eucalyptus oil with a carrier oil such as jojoba or coconut oil and use it as a moisturizer for dry or irritated skin.

- Add a few drops of eucalyptus oil to your shampoo or conditioner to promote healthy hair growth and improve scalp health.

- Mix a few drops of eucalyptus oil with water and use it as a natural toner to help tighten pores and reduce inflammation.

- Conclusion Eucalyptus oil is a versatile and natural

remedy that can be used for a wide range of practical purposes, from aromatherapy to household cleaning to skincare. Incorporating eucalyptus oil into your daily routine can provide a host of benefits and help promote overall health and wellness.

CHAPTER THREE

How to Use Eucalyptus Oil

Eucalyptus oil has numerous health benefits, but it's important to use it safely and effectively. In this chapter, we will discuss the various ways to use eucalyptus oil, including topical application, inhalation, and ingestion. We will also provide tips on how to use eucalyptus oil safely and effectively.

Topical Application

Topical application involves applying eucalyptus oil directly to the skin. It can be used to relieve muscle pain, joint pain, and skin conditions such as acne, psoriasis, and eczema. Here are some tips for using eucalyptus oil topically:

Dilute eucalyptus oil with a carrier oil, such as coconut oil or almond oil, before applying it to the skin. This will help prevent skin irritation or allergic reactions.

Always do a patch test before using eucalyptus oil on a larger area of skin. Apply a small amount of diluted eucalyptus oil to the inside of your wrist and wait for 24 hours. If you experience any itching, redness, or swelling, do not use eucalyptus oil topically.

Apply eucalyptus oil to the affected area and massage it gently into the skin. Do not apply eucalyptus oil to broken skin, wounds, or sensitive areas such as the eyes or genitals.

Wash your hands thoroughly after applying eucalyptus oil topically to prevent accidental ingestion or irritation to other parts of your body.

Inhalation

Inhalation involves breathing in eucalyptus oil vapor. It can be used to relieve respiratory problems such as coughs, colds, and sinusitis. Here are some tips for inhaling eucalyptus oil:

Add a few drops of eucalyptus oil to a bowl of hot water and inhale the steam for 5-10 minutes. You can also add eucalyptus oil to a diffuser or humidifier and breathe in the vapor.

Do not inhale eucalyptus oil directly from the bottle, as this can irritate your nose, throat, and lungs.

Be careful not to overdo it when inhaling eucalyptus oil. Too much inhalation can cause headaches, nausea, and dizziness.

Ingestion

Ingestion involves consuming eucalyptus oil orally. It can be used to relieve digestive problems such as bloating, constipation, and indigestion. However, ingesting eucalyptus oil is not recommended for everyone and should be done under the guidance of a healthcare professional. Here are some tips for ingesting eucalyptus oil:

- Always use high-quality, pure eucalyptus oil that is

safe for ingestion. Do not ingest eucalyptus oil that is meant for topical or inhalation use.

- Start with a small amount of eucalyptus oil, such as 1-2 drops, and mix it with a carrier oil or honey to dilute it.

- Do not ingest eucalyptus oil if you are pregnant, breastfeeding, or have a history of seizures or liver disease.

- Consult a healthcare professional before ingesting eucalyptus oil if you are taking any medications or have any health conditions.

Safety Precautions

Eucalyptus oil is generally safe when used as directed, but it can cause side effects in some people. Here are some safety precautions to keep in mind when using eucalyptus oil:

1. Do not use eucalyptus oil on children under the age of 2, as it can cause breathing difficulties and other adverse reactions.

2. Do not use eucalyptus oil if you are allergic to it or other members of the Myrtaceae

family, such as tea tree or clove.

3. Avoid using eucalyptus oil near the face, especially the nose and mouth, as it can cause irritation or breathing difficulties.

4. Keep eucalyptus oil out of reach of children and pets, as ingestion can cause serious health problems.

5. Store eucalyptus oil in a cool, dark place away from heat and sunlight, as it can degrade over time.

6. Always use eucalyptus oil according to the instructions

on the label or as directed by a healthcare professional.

In conclusion, eucalyptus oil is a versatile natural remedy with many health benefits. However, it's important to use it safely and effectively. Topical application, inhalation, and ingestion are the three main ways to use eucalyptus oil, but each method requires specific precautions and guidelines to ensure safety. By following these tips, you can unleash the healing power of eucalyptus oil while minimizing the risk of adverse reactions.

Homemade Chest Rub

Eucalyptus oil is a natural decongestant and can help to relieve respiratory problems such as coughs, colds, and bronchitis. A homemade chest rub using eucalyptus oil can be an effective way to soothe and alleviate symptoms.

Ingredients:

- 1/4 cup coconut oil
- 10 drops eucalyptus oil
- 10 drops peppermint oil
- 5 drops lavender oil

Instructions:

Melt the coconut oil in a double boiler or microwave.

- Remove from heat and add the eucalyptus, peppermint, and lavender oils.
- Stir well to combine.
- Transfer the mixture to a clean, airtight jar.
- Rub a small amount of the chest rub on your chest and neck as needed.

Natural Insect Repellent

Eucalyptus oil is a natural insect repellent and can be used to repel mosquitoes, ticks, and other biting insects. This DIY recipe is easy to make and can be a safer alternative to commercial insect repellents that may contain harmful chemicals.

Ingredients:

- 1/4 cup witch hazel
- 1/4 cup apple cider vinegar
- 10 drops eucalyptus oil
- 10 drops lemon oil
- 5 drops peppermint oil

Instructions:

- Combine the witch hazel and apple cider vinegar in a spray bottle.

- Add the eucalyptus, lemon, and peppermint oils.
- Shake well to combine.
- Spray the insect repellent on your skin before going outdoors.

Homemade Household Cleaner

Eucalyptus oil is a natural antiseptic and can be used as a cleaning agent around the home. This DIY recipe is a safe and effective way to clean and disinfect surfaces.

Ingredients:

- 1/2 cup white vinegar

- 1/2 cup water
- 10 drops eucalyptus oil
- 10 drops tea tree oil

Instructions:

- Combine the white vinegar and water in a spray bottle.
- Add the eucalyptus and tea tree oils.
- Shake well to combine.
- Spray the cleaning solution on surfaces and wipe clean with a cloth.

Benefits of DIY Eucalyptus Oil Recipes

- There are many benefits to making your own eucalyptus

oil recipes. First, you can control the quality of the ingredients and ensure that you are using natural, safe products. Commercial products often contain harmful chemicals that can be harmful to your health and the environment.

- Second, DIY recipes can save you money in the long run. Many commercial products are expensive, and you may need to buy them repeatedly. By making your own eucalyptus oil recipes, you can save money and reduce your environmental impact.

- Finally, making your own eucalyptus oil recipes can be a fun and rewarding experience. You can experiment with different ingredients and find the perfect recipe for your needs. Additionally, you can customize your recipes to suit your preferences and avoid ingredients that you may be allergic to or sensitive to.

DIY eucalyptus oil recipes are a safe, effective, and affordable way to incorporate the healing power of nature into your daily life.

Whether you are looking to relieve respiratory problems, repel insects, or clean your home, there is a DIY eucalyptus oil recipe for you.

By using natural ingredients and avoiding harmful chemicals, you can promote a healthier and more sustainable lifestyle. Making your own products can also be a fun and creative way to explore the benefits of eucalyptus oil and other natural remedies.

Remember to always use high-quality, pure essential oils and to follow safety precautions when using them. Additionally, it's important to test a small amount of any DIY product on your skin before using it more widely to ensure that you do not have an adverse reaction.

Incorporating eucalyptus oil into your daily routine can help to unleash the healing power of nature and promote a healthier, more sustainable lifestyle. With these DIY recipes, you can explore the many benefits of eucalyptus oil and create natural products that are safe, effective, and affordable.

CHAPTER FOUR

The Benefits of Natural Remedies

The use of natural remedies dates back to ancient times, and with good reason. Natural remedies like eucalyptus oil offer a variety of benefits over commercial products that may contain harmful chemicals. Natural remedies are often safer and more effective than their synthetic counterparts, and they are typically more affordable as well.

In addition to their health benefits, natural remedies also have a lower environmental impact than commercial products. Many commercial products are made with harsh chemicals that can harm the environment and wildlife, but natural remedies like eucalyptus oil are biodegradable and non-toxic.

Incorporating Eucalyptus Oil into Your Daily Life

Now that we have explored the benefits of natural remedies like eucalyptus oil, it's important to discuss how to incorporate them into your daily life. There are many ways to use eucalyptus oil, from adding a few drops to your diffuser to creating your own homemade cleaning products.

One easy way to incorporate eucalyptus oil into your daily routine is through aromatherapy. Simply add a few drops of eucalyptus oil to a diffuser or humidifier to enjoy its relaxing and rejuvenating effects. You can also add a few drops of eucalyptus oil to your bath for a soothing and refreshing experience.

Eucalyptus oil can also be used topically for a variety of purposes. It can be added to carrier oils like coconut oil or jojoba oil and used as a massage oil to relieve sore muscles and joints. It can also be added to skincare products like lotions and balms to soothe dry, irritated skin.

In addition to its therapeutic uses, eucalyptus oil can also be used in household cleaning. It has natural antiseptic properties that make it an effective alternative to commercial cleaning products. You can create your own all-purpose cleaner by adding a few drops of eucalyptus oil to water and vinegar.

Safety Considerations

While eucalyptus oil is generally safe to use, there are a few safety considerations to keep in mind. It should not be ingested, as it can be toxic in large amounts. It should also be used with caution on the skin, as it can cause irritation in some people. It's always a good idea to do a patch test before using eucalyptus oil topically.

Conclusion

Eucalyptus oil is a powerful and versatile natural remedy that offers a variety of health and household benefits. By incorporating eucalyptus oil into your daily routine, you can enjoy its therapeutic properties and reduce your reliance on synthetic products. Whether you're using it for aromatherapy, skincare, or cleaning, eucalyptus oil is a valuable addition to any natural wellness toolkit.

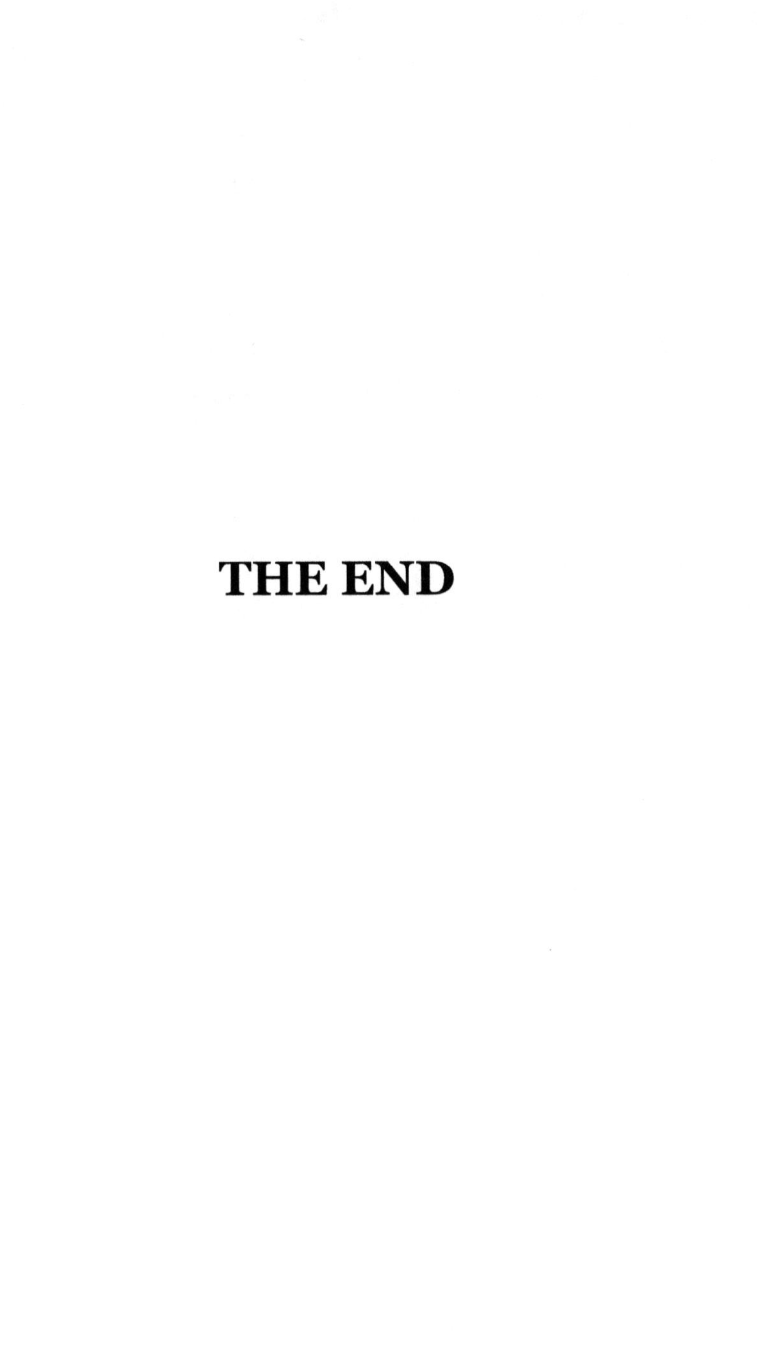

THE END